Yoga for Beginners

A Complete Step-by-Step Self-Practice Guide to Simple Yoga Poses and Breathing Exercises to Calm the Mind, Relieve Stress, Strengthen the Body, and Increase Flexibility

Mind, Body, and Spirit Masterclass

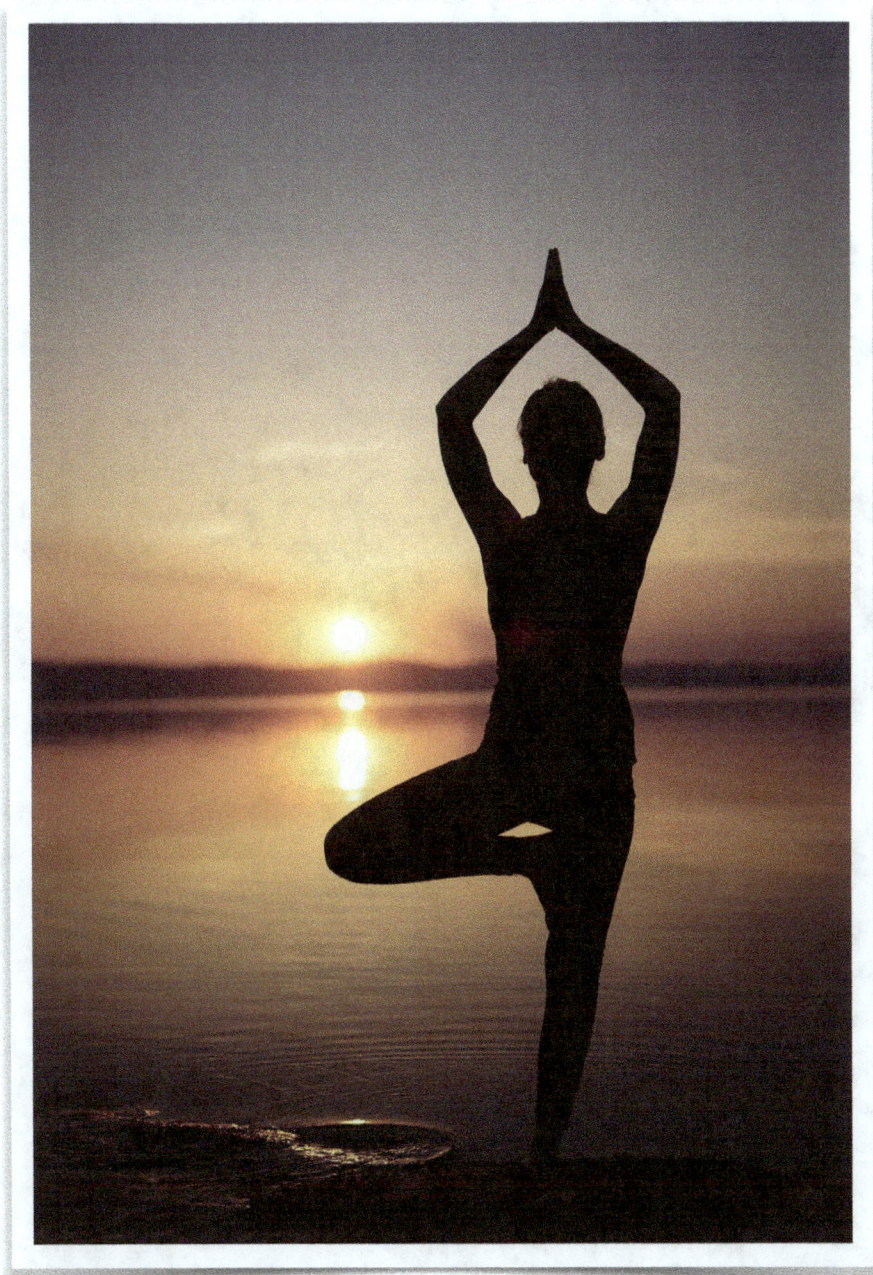

© Copyright 2023 - Mind, Body, and Spirit Masterclass - All rights reserved.

The following Book is reproduced below with the goal of providing information that is as accurate and reliable as possible. Regardless, purchasing this Book can be seen as consent to the fact that both the publisher and the author of this book are in no way experts on the topics discussed within and that any recommendations or suggestions that are made herein are for entertainment purposes only. Professionals should be consulted as needed prior to undertaking any of the action endorsed herein.

This declaration is deemed fair and valid by both the American Bar Association and the Committee of Publishers Association and is legally binding throughout the United States.

Furthermore, the transmission, duplication, or reproduction of any of the following work including specific information will be considered an illegal act irrespective of if it is done electronically or in print. This extends to creating a secondary or tertiary copy of the work or a recorded copy and is only allowed with the express written consent from the Publisher. All additional right reserved.

The information in the following pages is broadly considered a truthful and accurate account of facts and as such, any inattention, use, or misuse of the information in question by the reader will render any resulting actions solely under their purview. There are no scenarios in which the publisher or the original author of this work can be in any fashion deemed liable for any hardship or damages that may befall them after undertaking information described herein.

Additionally, the information in the following pages is intended only for informational purposes and should thus be thought of as universal. As befitting its nature, it is presented without assurance regarding its prolonged validity or interim quality. Trademarks that are mentioned are done without written consent and can in no way be considered an endorsement from the trademark holder.

Table of Contents

Introduction
11

What is Yoga?
11

Benefits of Yoga
13

Types of Yoga
15

Choosing the Right Yoga Style
18

Chapter 1: Yoga Philosophy and Spirituality
21

The Origins and History of Yoga
21

The Yoga Sutras of Patanjali
22

The Eight Limbs of Yoga
23

Meditation and Yoga
25

Yoga and Religion
27

Chapter 2: Getting Started
29

Equipment and Clothing
29

Setting Up Your Space
32

Basic Yoga Positions
35

Standing Poses
35

Sitting Poses
37

Lying-Down Poses
38

Inversions
39

Cool-Down Poses
41

The Foundations
43

Breathing Techniques
48

Building a Yoga Routine
51

Including Yoga Into Your Workout Routine
53

Incorporating Yoga Into Your Daily Life
54

Chapter 3: Yoga for Health and Wellness
57

Yoga for Stress Relief
57

Yoga for Flexibility and Strength
60

Yoga for Cardiovascular Health
65

Yoga for Mental Health
75

Yoga for Weight Management
78

Chapter 4: Yoga for Special Populations
81

Yoga for Seniors
81

Yoga for Children
83

Yoga for Pregnant Women
85

Yoga for Athletes
87

Yoga for People with Chronic Conditions
89

Chapter 5: Misunderstandings and False Beliefs About Yoga
91

Conclusion
95

Tips for a Successful Yoga Practice
95

Warnings
96

Glossary of Yoga Terms
98

The Path to Total Wellness & Recommended Reading
99

Introduction

Welcome to "Yoga for Beginners"! This book is designed to help you start your yoga journey and develop a regular practice that will benefit your body, mind, and spirit.

What is Yoga?

Yoga is an ancient practice that originated in India more than 5,000 years ago. It is a holistic system of self-care and spiritual practices that combines physical postures, breathing exercises, and meditation. Yoga is not just a physical exercise, but a way of life that promotes balance, harmony, and well-being.

The word "yoga" comes from the Sanskrit word "yuj" which means "to unite or join." The ultimate goal of yoga is to unite the individual self with the universal self, or the individual consciousness with the divine consciousness.

Yoga has been practiced for thousands of years. It encompasses a wide range of physical, mental, and spiritual techniques and is designed to bring balance and harmony to the body, mind, and spirit.

At its core, yoga is a practice of physical postures (asanas), controlled breathing (pranayama), and meditation (dhyana). Through these practices, yoga aims to strengthen the body, calm the mind, and increase awareness and connection to the present moment.

In addition to its physical benefits, yoga is also considered a spiritual discipline that seeks to promote inner peace, self-awareness, and a sense of unity with all things. Many people who practice yoga report feeling more relaxed, focused, and energized after their practice, and experience long-term benefits such as improved flexibility, strength, and mental clarity.

Overall, yoga is a multi-faceted practice that offers a wide range of benefits and can be adapted to suit the individual needs and goals of each practitioner. Whether you are looking to improve your physical health, reduce stress, or deepen your spiritual connection, yoga can be a valuable tool to help you on your journey.

Benefits of Yoga

Yoga offers a wide range of benefits, both physical and mental. Regular yoga practice can improve flexibility, strength, balance, and cardiovascular health. It can also help reduce stress, anxiety, and depression, and improve sleep and overall well-being. Yoga can also be helpful for specific health conditions such as lower back pain, asthma, and diabetes.

Here are some of the major benefits of practicing yoga:

1. **Improved flexibility and strength:** Yoga requires you to move your body through a range of motions, which can help to increase flexibility and strength over time.

2. **Reduced stress and anxiety:** Many yoga poses and breathing techniques are designed to calm the mind and reduce stress and anxiety.

3. **Better posture:** Many yoga poses help to improve posture by strengthening the muscles that support the spine.

4. **Improved balance and coordination:** Yoga requires you to balance and coordinate your movements, which can help to improve these skills over time.

5. **Better sleep:** Yoga has been shown to improve sleep quality, which can help you feel more rested and refreshed.

6. **Better breathing:** Yoga emphasizes the importance of breathing and teaches techniques to help you breathe more deeply and efficiently.

7. **Increased focus and concentration:** Yoga requires focus and concentration, which can help to improve these skills over time.

8. **Better overall physical health:** Practicing yoga regularly has been shown to have a positive impact on a range of physical health conditions, such as heart disease, high blood pressure, and chronic pain.

These are just a few examples of the many benefits that yoga can offer. Of course, everyone's experience with yoga will be unique, and the benefits you experience will depend on a range of factors, such as your goals, the type of yoga you practice, and how frequently you practice.

Types of Yoga

There are many different styles of yoga, each with its own unique focus, style, and approach. Each style offers different benefits and is suitable for different levels of fitness and experience.

Some of the most common types of yoga include:

1. **Hatha Yoga:** Hatha yoga is a general term that is often used to describe any type of yoga that involves physical postures. Hatha yoga is a great starting point for beginners, as it is a gentle form of yoga that focuses on holding poses for a longer period of time.

2. **Vinyasa Yoga:** Vinyasa yoga is a type of yoga that emphasizes flow and movement, with each movement linked to a breath. Vinyasa yoga is a more active form of yoga that can be a good choice for those looking for a more vigorous workout.

3. **Iyengar Yoga:** Iyengar yoga is a type of yoga that focuses on precision and alignment, using props such as blocks and straps to help practitioners hold poses more effectively.

4. **Ashtanga Yoga:** Ashtanga yoga is a dynamic and physically demanding form of yoga that involves a set sequence of postures performed in a specific order.

5. **Bikram Yoga:** Bikram yoga is a type of hot yoga that is practiced in a room that is heated to 105°F (40°C) with a humidity of 40%. Bikram yoga is a physically demanding form of yoga that is known for its ability to help practitioners detoxify and sweat out impurities.

6. **Kundalini Yoga:** Kundalini yoga is a type of yoga that focuses on awakening the dormant energy at the base of the spine and raising it up through the chakras to the crown of the head. Kundalini yoga is a spiritual form of yoga that combines physical postures, breathing techniques, and meditation.

7. **Restorative Yoga:** Restorative yoga is a type of yoga that focuses on using props to support the body in poses that are held for a longer period of time. Restorative yoga is a gentle form of yoga that is designed to help practitioners relax and restore their energy.

8. **Yin yoga:** A slow-paced form of yoga that emphasizes passive stretching and the holding of postures for extended periods of time to release tension in the body.

These are just a few examples of the many different types of yoga that are practiced today. The type of yoga that is right for you will depend on your goals, preferences, and physical abilities, so it's important to try out different types of yoga to see what works best for you.

At this point, you are probably asking yourself: "So what kind of yoga covers the poses I am learning in this book?".

The various poses I will cover in this book can be found in a variety of yoga styles, including Hatha yoga, Vinyasa yoga, Ashtanga yoga, and many others. These poses are generally considered foundational poses in yoga, as they help to build strength, stability, and flexibility in the body.

In Hatha yoga, for example, you might practice standing poses such as Warrior I (Virabhadrasana I) or Triangle Pose (Trikonasana), and sitting poses such as Seated Forward Bend (Paschimottanasana) or Lotus Pose (Padmasana). In Vinyasa yoga, you might flow through sequences of standing and sitting poses as part of a dynamic and flowing practice.

Basically, the different types of yoga may place different emphasis on different poses and may incorporate different variations or modifications of the same pose. However, many of the foundational standing, sitting, or other kinds of poses are commonly found across different styles of yoga and are a great starting point for anyone new to yoga.

Choosing the Right Yoga Style

When choosing a yoga style, it is important to consider your personal preferences, physical abilities, fitness level, and health conditions. It may be helpful to try a few different styles to see which one you prefer. It is also important to find a qualified teacher who can guide you through the correct alignment and modifications.

Here are some factors to consider when choosing the best type of yoga for you:

1. **Physical abilities:** Consider your current fitness level and any physical limitations you may have. Some forms of yoga, such as vinyasa or ashtanga, are more physically demanding, while others, such as Hatha or restorative yoga, are more gentle.

2. **Goals:** Consider what you hope to get out of your yoga practice. Do you want to improve your physical strength and flexibility, reduce stress and anxiety, or explore the spiritual aspects of yoga? Different types of yoga will emphasize different aspects of the practice, so choose one that aligns with your goals.

3. **Schedule and availability:** Consider the time you have available for your yoga practice and where you would like to practice. Some types of yoga, such as Bikram or hot yoga, require a specific environment, while

others, such as vinyasa or ashtanga, can be practiced in a variety of settings.

4. **Personal preferences:** Consider your personal preferences, such as the pace of the class, the type of music or atmosphere, and the style of teaching. Some people prefer a more slow-paced and meditative approach, while others enjoy a more vigorous and energetic practice.

It's also a good idea to try out a few different types of yoga to see what works best for you. Most yoga studios offer a variety of classes, so you can try out different types of yoga to find the one that feels right for you, before proceeding on your own if you prefer. Additionally, there are many online resources, such as videos and tutorials, that can help you explore different types of yoga from the comfort of your own home.

I hope this book will inspire you to start your yoga journey and discover the many benefits it has to offer. With regular practice, you will see improvements in your physical, mental, and emotional well-being. Happy reading and happy yoga!

Chapter 1: Yoga Philosophy and Spirituality

The Origins and History of Yoga

Yoga is an ancient practice that has its roots in India and has been around for thousands of years. It's difficult to determine exactly when yoga began, but it is believed to have originated between 5,000 and 10,000 years ago.

The early texts of yoga, known as the Vedas, suggest that yoga was originally developed as a spiritual discipline aimed at attaining union with the divine. Over time, yoga evolved and was systematized into various philosophical schools, each with its own interpretation of the teachings and practices of yoga.

One of the earliest and most influential texts on yoga is the "Yoga Sutras of Patanjali," which was written by the sage Patanjali in the 2nd century BCE. The Yoga Sutras outline the eight limbs of yoga, which form the framework for the practice of yoga and include moral and ethical codes, physical postures, breathing techniques, and meditation.

In the centuries that followed, yoga continued to evolve and develop into the various forms that we know today and that I listed in the "Introduction", such as Hatha Yoga, Kundalini Yoga, and Ashtanga Yoga, to name just a few. In recent decades, yoga has become increasingly popular around the world as a means of exercise and stress relief, as well as for its spiritual and philosophical elements.

The Yoga Sutras of Patanjali

The Yoga Sutras of Patanjali is an ancient text that lays out the principles of yoga. It is considered to be one of the most important texts on yoga and is still widely studied today.

It was written by the sage Patanjali in the 2nd century BCE and is considered to be one of the foundational texts of yoga. The text consists of 195 sutras, or brief aphorisms, that outline the teachings and practices of yoga and provide guidance for living a yogic lifestyle.

The "Yoga Sutras of Patanjali" is organized into four chapters, with each chapter addressing a different aspect of yoga. The first chapter, Samadhi Pada, discusses the nature of the mind and the path to spiritual enlightenment. The second chapter, Sadhana Pada, outlines the practices of yoga, including the eight limbs of yoga, and their role in the path to enlightenment. The third chapter, Vibhuti Pada, focuses on the mystical powers that may arise from the practice of yoga, while the fourth chapter, Kaivalya Pada, discusses the ultimate goal of yoga and the state of liberation.

The "Yoga Sutras of Patanjali" is considered to be one of the most important texts in the history of yoga and is still widely studied and referenced by yoga practitioners and teachers today. Its teachings continue to influence and inspire modern interpretations of yoga and are considered a valuable source of wisdom and guidance for those seeking to deepen their practice and understanding of yoga.

The Eight Limbs of Yoga

The eight limbs of yoga, as described in the "Yoga Sutras of Patanjali," are a set of guidelines for living a yogic lifestyle, a comprehensive framework for the practice of yoga, and serve as a roadmap for spiritual development. The eight limbs are:

1. **Yama:** ethical guidelines for behavior towards others. This limb encompasses the ethical and moral codes of conduct and includes five principles: non-violence, truthfulness, non-stealing, non-excess, and non-possessiveness.

2. **Niyama:** ethical guidelines for behavior towards oneself. This limb involves personal observances and practices, such as cleanliness, contentment, self-discipline, self-study, and surrender to a higher power.

3. **Asana:** physical postures. This limb refers to the physical postures and poses that are commonly associated with yoga. The purpose of these postures is to cultivate strength, flexibility, and stability in the body.

4. **Pranayama:** breath control. This limb involves the control and regulation of the breath, which is considered to be the source of life energy or prana. Pranayama practices are intended to help calm the mind, increase energy, and promote overall health.

5. **Pratyahara:** withdrawal of the senses. This limb involves withdrawing the senses from external stimuli and turning inward towards the self. It is considered the first step in the development of concentration and meditation.

6. **Dharana:** concentration. This limb involves concentration and the ability to focus the mind on a single point or object. This is the foundation for developing deeper levels of meditation.

7. **Dhyana:** meditation. This limb involves deep meditation and the experience of unity and connection with the divine. It is described as a state of continuous and effortless concentration.

8. **Samadhi:** the state of unity with the divine. This limb represents the highest state of consciousness and enlightenment, in which the individual experiences a sense of unity with the divine and all of existence.

These eight limbs work together to provide a comprehensive approach to yoga that transcends the physical practice and encompasses the spiritual, ethical, and psychological aspects of the practice as well.

Meditation and Yoga

Meditation is an integral part of yoga practice. It is the process of calming the mind and focusing attention. There are many different types of meditation, including mindfulness meditation, transcendental meditation, and yoga nidra.

In many styles of yoga, meditation is integrated into the practice as a whole and is often included at the beginning or end of a yoga session as a time for stillness and introspection. For example, some forms of yoga include pranayama, or breath control, which can help to calm the mind and prepare the practitioner for meditation.

Yoga Nidra, on the other hand, is a specific type of meditation that is practiced lying down or seated comfortably and is often referred to as "yogic sleep." The practice involves systematically relaxing each part of the body and calming the mind through guided visualization and awareness of the breath. The goal of Yoga Nidra is to achieve a state of deep relaxation and to experience a sense of inner peace and rejuvenation.

Meditation is an integral part of the practice of yoga, and Yoga Nidra is a specific form of meditation that is often used in yoga to help calm the mind and relax the body. Both practices aim to cultivate inner peace, reduce stress, and promote overall well-being.

Yoga and mindfulness meditation are deeply interconnected practices that can complement each other in many ways, too.

1. **Yoga as a physical expression of mindfulness:** Many yoga postures and sequences are designed to bring your focus to the present moment, and to help you tune into your body, breath, and surroundings. This physical expression of mindfulness can help you cultivate greater awareness and focus in your daily life.

2. **Mindfulness as a foundation for yoga:** Mindfulness is a key component of many yoga practices, and is often emphasized in the yoga sutras of Patanjali. By bringing your attention to the present moment, mindfulness can help you deepen your yoga practice and get more out of your poses.

3. **Yoga and mindfulness for stress reduction:** Both yoga and mindfulness have been shown to be effective tools for reducing stress and improving mental health. Practicing yoga and mindfulness together can help you manage stress and improve your overall well-being.

4. **Integration of yoga and mindfulness in daily life:** By integrating yoga and mindfulness into your daily life, you can develop greater awareness, focus, and relaxation, and cultivate a more positive outlook. This can help you live with greater intention and purpose, and bring more peace and happiness into your life.

Yoga and mindfulness are two powerful practices that can enhance each other and bring many benefits to your life. Whether you practice yoga as a physical expression of mindfulness or use mindfulness to deepen your yoga practice, incorporating both into your daily routine can help you cultivate greater awareness, focus, and well-being.

Yoga and Religion

Yoga is not a religion but rather a spiritual practice that can be used to enhance one's religious beliefs. Yoga is compatible with most major religions, including Christianity, Judaism, Islam, and Buddhism.

Yoga philosophy and spirituality can provide a deeper understanding and connection to the practice and can be beneficial to those seeking a more holistic approach to self-care. Remember that the practice should be tailored to one's own beliefs and preferences, and it should not be forced upon anyone.

Chapter 2: Getting Started

Equipment and Clothing

For yoga, you don't need much equipment, a comfortable yoga mat is the only essential piece of equipment. Yoga props such as blocks, straps, blankets, and bolsters can also be helpful, but they are not necessary for beginners, especially if you are not yet sure you will carry on with the practice. When it comes to clothing, it is best to wear comfortable, stretchy clothing that allows you to move freely. Avoid clothes that are too tight or restrictive.

However, as you go on with practice and you have decided to stick with it, it's important to have the right clothing and equipment to ensure that you are comfortable and able to perform the postures and movements correctly. Here are some basic suggestions:

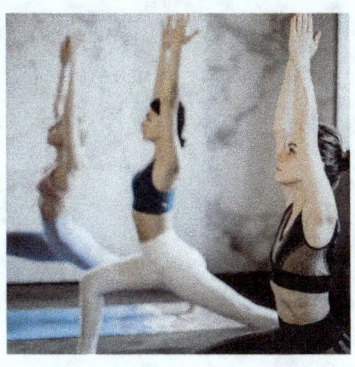

1.**Clothing:** Choose comfortable, form-fitting clothing that allows you to move freely and does not restrict your movements. Stretchy fabric like cotton or bamboo is ideal for yoga practice. Avoid wearing loose clothing as it may get in the way during certain postures.

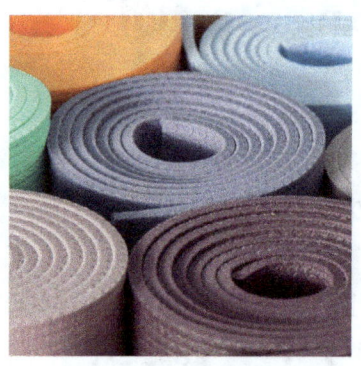

2.**Mat:** A yoga mat provides a non-slip surface to practice on and helps to cushion your joints during postures. Look for a mat that is the right thickness and texture for your needs, and consider the material and durability of the mat as well.

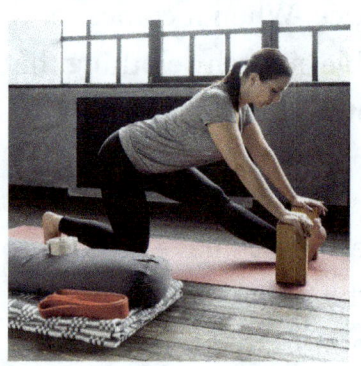

3.**Props:** Depending on your needs and preferences, you may find that props such as blocks, straps, blankets, or bolsters can help you to perform postures more effectively and safely.

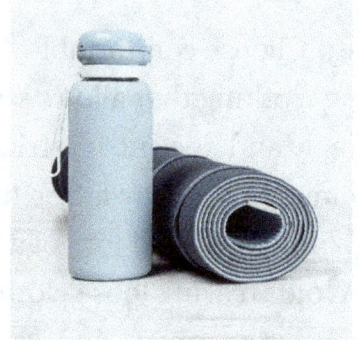

4.**Water:** It's important to stay hydrated during your yoga practice, so bring a water bottle with you.

It's also a good idea to bring a towel and to wear a comfortable pair of shoes to and from your yoga practice, as well as any other items you may need for personal hygiene or comfort.

In conclusion, the most important thing is to feel comfortable and supported in your practice, so you can fully focus on your breathing and movements.

Setting Up Your Space

You can practice yoga anywhere, whether it's in a dedicated yoga studio, at home, or in a park. It is important to find a quiet, distraction-free space where you can focus on your practice. Make sure your space is well-ventilated and has enough room for you to move around freely.

However, setting up a space for your yoga practice at home can help you create a dedicated and supportive environment for your practice. I mostly practice at home (or open air when the weather allows it) that's why I find it very important to have a yoga space at home. In my case, it's the same space I use for meditation and chakras' healing.

Here are some tips for creating a yoga space in your home:

1. **Location:** Choose a quiet and peaceful area of your home where you will not be disturbed during your practice. If possible, find a space that gets natural light and has good ventilation.

2. **Mat:** Unroll your yoga mat and place it in the center of your space. Make sure it is flat and even and that there is enough space around it for you to move freely in all directions.

3. **Props:** Keep your yoga props, such as blocks, straps, blankets, and bolsters, within easy reach so that you can easily access them during your practice.

4. **Lighting:** If possible, choose a location with natural light and make sure that the room is well-lit. If you need additional lighting, use soft, indirect lighting to create a calm and peaceful atmosphere.

5. **Decor:** You can create a calming atmosphere in your yoga space by adding plants, candles, or other decorative elements that you find relaxing and peaceful.

6. **Noise reduction:** If necessary, use earplugs or a white noise machine to reduce any distracting sounds.

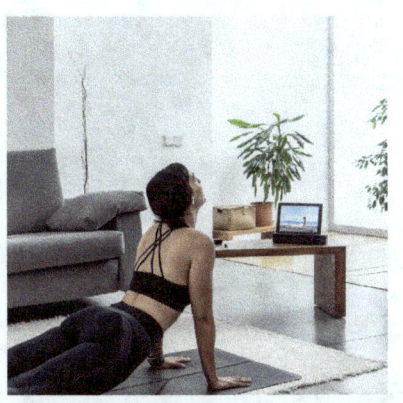
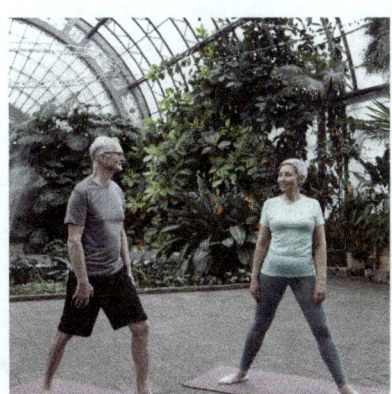
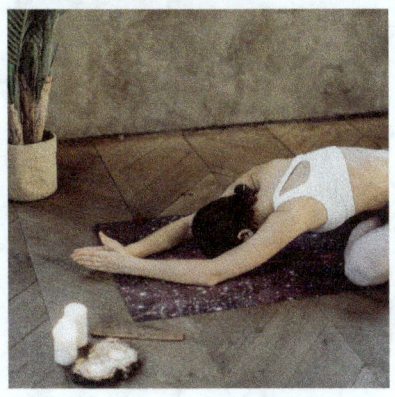
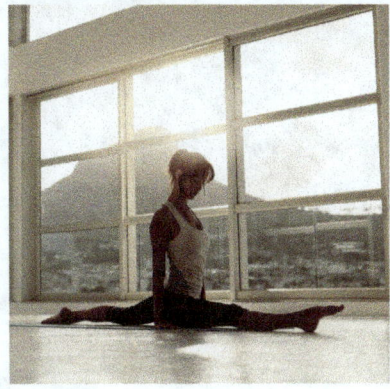

In conclusion, creating a dedicated yoga space in your home can help you create a supportive environment for your practice and allow you to fully focus on your breath and movements. The most important thing is to make your space comfortable and relaxing so that you can fully immerse yourself in your practice.

Basic Yoga Positions

Before starting your practice, it is important to learn the basic yoga positions (or postures, or poses).

Yoga poses are usually divided into 5 groups for practical reasons. Those groups are:

- Standing Poses
- Sitting Poses
- Lying Down Poses
- Inversions
- Cool-Down Poses

Standing Poses

Standing yoga poses are an essential part of many yoga practices and are typically used to build strength, improve balance and stability, and increase flexibility in the legs and hips. Some of the most commonly practiced standing yoga poses include:

1. Mountain Pose (Tadasana): This pose strengthens the legs, improves posture, and helps to calm the mind.

2. Warrior I (Virabhadrasana I): This pose strengthens the legs, hips, and core, and also improves balance and stability.

3. Warrior II (Virabhadrasana II): This pose strengthens the legs, hips, and core, and also opens up the hips and chest.

4. Triangle Pose (Trikonasana): This pose strengthens the legs and hips, and also stretches the hips, hamstrings, and sides of the waist.

5. Tree Pose (Vrksasana): This pose improves balance and stability, and strengthens the legs, hips, and core.

6. Downward-Facing Dog (Adho Mukha Svanasana): This pose strengthens the arms, legs, and spine, and also improves flexibility in the hamstrings, calves, and hips.

7. Half Moon Pose (Ardha Chandrasana): This pose strengthens the legs, hips, and core, and also improves balance and stability.

8. Chair Pose (Utkatasana): This pose strengthens the legs, hips, and core, and also improves balance and stability.

These are just a few examples of standing yoga poses. There are many others to explore as well, and practicing a variety of standing poses can help you build strength, improve balance and stability, and increase flexibility in your legs and hips.

Sitting Poses

Sitting yoga poses are an important part of many yoga practices and are typically used to improve flexibility, release tension, and calm the mind. Some of the most commonly practiced sitting yoga poses include:

1. Easy Pose (Sukhasana): This pose is a simple seated posture that is great for meditation and breathing practices.

2. Seated Forward Bend (Paschimottanasana): This pose stretches the hamstrings, hips, and lower back, and can help to calm the mind.

3. Cobbler's Pose (Baddha Konasana): This pose opens up the hips and groin, and can help to release tension in the lower back and hips.

4. Bound Angle Pose (Baddha Konasana): This pose opens up the hips and groin, and can also help to calm the mind.

5. Hero Pose (Virasana): This pose strengthens the legs and knees, and can also help to release tension in the hips and lower back.

6. Half Lotus Pose (Ardha Padmasana): This pose is often used in meditation and breathing practices, and can help to improve flexibility in the hips and knees.

7. Lotus Pose (Padmasana): This pose is often used in meditation and breathing practices, and can help to improve flexibility in the hips and knees.

These are just a few examples of sitting yoga poses. There are many others to explore as well, and practicing a variety of sitting poses can help you improve flexibility, release tension, and calm the mind. Additionally, many sitting poses are great for preparing the body and mind for meditation, making them an important part of many yoga practices.

Lying-Down Poses

Lying-down yoga poses, also known as supine poses, are an important part of many yoga practices and are typically used to stretch the muscles, release tension, and calm the mind. Some of the most commonly practiced lying-down yoga poses include:

1. Corpse Pose (Savasana): This pose is a simple lying down pose that is often used to close a yoga practice, allowing the body and mind to fully relax.

2. Bridge Pose (Setu Bandha Sarvangasana): This pose strengthens the spine, hips, and glutes, and also helps to release tension in the lower back.

3. Shoulder Stand (Sarvangasana): This pose strengthens the spine, neck, and shoulders, and also helps to improve circulation and digestion.

4. Fish Pose (Matsyasana): This pose opens up the chest and throat, and also helps to release tension in the neck and shoulders.

5. Happy Baby Pose (Ananda Balasana): This pose releases tension in the hips and lower back, and can also be used to calm the mind.

6. Spinal Twist (Jathara Parivartanasana): This pose helps to stretch the spine, hips, and back, and can also improve digestion and circulation.

These are just a few examples of lying-down yoga poses. There are many others to explore as well, and practicing a variety of lying-down poses can help you stretch the muscles, release tension, and calm the mind. Additionally, many lying-down poses are great for preparing the body and mind for meditation, making them an important part of many yoga practices.

Inversions

Inversions are yoga poses where the head is below the heart, which can have a number of benefits for the body and mind. Some of the most commonly practiced inversion poses include:

1. Downward-Facing Dog (Adho Mukha Svanasana): This pose is a staple of many yoga practices and is a great way to stretch the legs, hips, and spine.

2. Headstand (Sirsasana): This pose strengthens the arms, shoulders, and core, and can also improve circulation and concentration.

3. Shoulder Stand (Sarvangasana): This pose strengthens the spine, neck, and shoulders, and also helps to improve circulation and digestion.

4. Handstand (Adho Mukha Vrksasana): This pose strengthens the arms, shoulders, and core, and can also improve balance and concentration.

5. Forearm Stand (Pincha Mayurasana): This pose strengthens the arms, shoulders, and core, and can also improve balance and concentration.

These are just a few examples of inversion poses. There are many others to explore as well, and practicing a variety of inversion poses can help you improve balance, strength, and concentration. However, it's important to note that inversions can be challenging, and they may not be appropriate for everyone, especially those with certain medical conditions. If you are new to yoga or have any concerns, it's best to speak with a teacher or healthcare provider before attempting these poses.

Cool-Down Poses

Cool-down poses, also known as relaxation or restorative poses, are an important part of any yoga practice, as they help to calm the mind and release tension in the body. Some of the most commonly practiced cool-down poses include:

1. Child's Pose (Balasana): This pose helps to release tension in the back, hips, and legs, and also calms the mind.

2. Legs up the Wall (Viparita Karani): This pose helps to reduce stress and tension in the legs, hips, and lower back, and also improves circulation.

3. Reclined Bound Angle Pose (Supta Baddha Konasana): This pose helps to release tension in the hips and inner thighs, and also calms the mind.

4. Corpse Pose (Savasana): This pose is a simple lying down pose that is often used to close a yoga practice, allowing the body and mind to fully relax.

5. Happy Baby Pose (Ananda Balasana): This pose releases tension in the hips and lower back, and can also be used to calm the mind.

These are just a few examples of cool-down poses. There are many others to explore as well, and incorporating a variety of cool-down poses into your practice can help you to calm the mind and release tension in the body. Additionally, cool-down poses are great for preparing the body and mind for meditation, making them an important part of many yoga practices.

I will describe the main ones in the next few chapters as we meet them, mostly organized by the best use of each pose, for example, stress relief, flexibility, or strength. They will also be illustrated by a picture of a person correctly performing each pose, so you will have a clear image of what a correct performance should look like.

The Foundations

The following poses are considered the foundations for more advanced poses and will help you develop proper alignment and balance.

Tadasana (Mountain Pose)

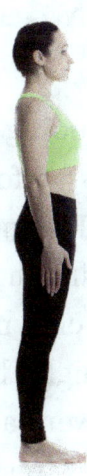

Tadasana, also known as mountain pose, is a standing pose in yoga. The pose is performed by standing upright with the feet together and the arms at the sides. The shoulders are relaxed and the spine is straight. The gaze is forward. The pose is often used as a starting position for other standing poses and can help to improve posture and balance.

Uttanasana (Standing Forward Bend)

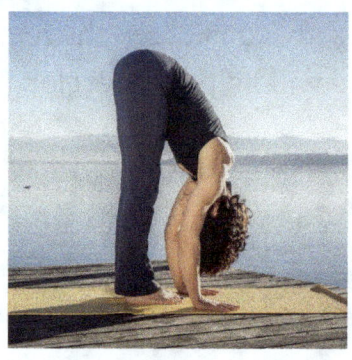

Uttanasana, also known as standing forward bend, is a forward-bending yoga pose. The pose is performed by standing upright with the feet hip-width apart. The individual then bends forward, with the aim of bringing their hands or fingers to the floor beside their feet, and the crown of the head towards the floor. The knees should be straight, but not locked. This pose can stretch the hamstrings, lower back, and spine. It can also calm the brain and help relieve stress and mild depression.

Adho Mukha Svanasana (Downward Facing Dog)

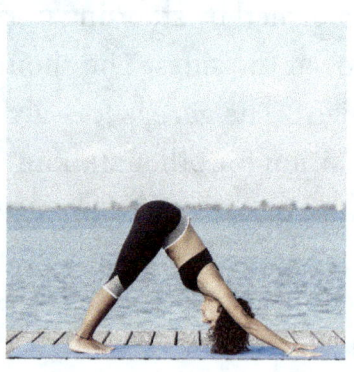

Adho Mukha Svanasana, also known as downward-facing dog, is a common yoga pose that resembles an inverted V-shape. The pose is performed by starting on your hands and knees with your wrists under your shoulders and your knees under your hips. Then, you lift your hips up and back, straightening your arms and legs, and coming into an inverted V-shape, with the head and heels reaching towards the floor. The gaze should be towards the navel. This pose can help to strengthen the arms, shoulders, and legs, and can also help to stretch the hamstrings, calves, and spine. It can also help to relieve stress and improve focus.

Urdhva Much Svanasana (Upward Facing Dog)

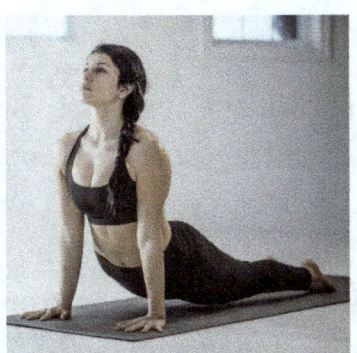

Urdhva Mukha Svanasana, also known as upward facing dog pose, is a common yoga pose. This pose is a back-bending yoga posture that is performed by starting in a prone position, with the tops of the feet on the floor, the hands placed beside the ribcage and the elbows close to the body. Then, lifting the chest and head up, straightening the arms, and engaging the legs and glutes to lift the body off the ground, creating a backbend. The gaze is towards the ceiling. This pose can help to strengthen the muscles of the back, arms, and legs, and also can help to stretch the chest, lungs, shoulders, and abdomen. It also helps to energize the whole body and improve posture.

Bhujangasana (Cobra Pose)

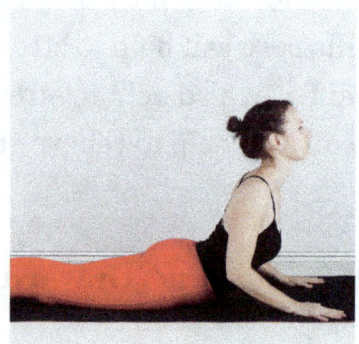

Bhujangasana, also known as Cobra Pose, is a yoga pose that resembles the raised hood of a cobra. The pose is performed by starting on your stomach with your hands next to your shoulders, and your elbows close to your body. Then, you press into your hands to lift your chest off the ground and back, straightening your arms and opening up the chest. The gaze should be towards the front. This pose can help to strengthen the muscles of the back, arms, and shoulders, and can also help to stretch the chest, lungs, and shoulders. It can also help to stimulate the abdominal organs and improve spinal flexibility. It's also said to have a positive effect on the nervous system and increase energy levels.

Savasana (Corpse Pose)

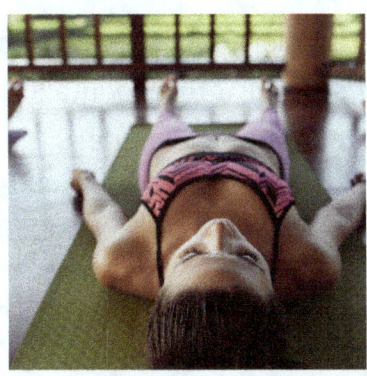

Savasana, also known as the corpse pose, is a yoga posture that is performed lying down on your back. It is often done at the end of a yoga practice to relax the body and mind.

To perform Savasana, lie on your back with your feet hip-width apart, and your arms resting by your side, with the palms facing up. Close your eyes, and allow your body to release any tension. Allow your breath to become slow and steady, and let go of any thoughts or distractions. The idea is to let the body and mind completely relax and reach a state of stillness. It's said that this pose can help to reduce stress and anxiety, improve sleep, and increase overall relaxation. It's also known as the 'final relaxation' pose, and it's often used as a way to end a yoga session.

Breathing Techniques

Breathing is an important aspect of yoga. It can help you focus and relax, and it can also have a therapeutic effect on your body. Some basic breathing techniques include:

Ujjayi breathing (Victorious Breath)

Ujjayi, also known as "victorious breath" or "ocean breath," is a pranayama (breathing technique) used in yoga. It is characterized by a slight contraction of the back of the throat, which creates a subtle sound or "ocean" like noise while inhaling and exhaling.

To practice Ujjayi breathing, sit in a comfortable position and take a deep breath in through your nose. Then, exhale through your nose while constricting the back of your throat, making the sound of the breath audible. The breath should be smooth and even, with no pauses or jerks. The breath should also be deep and long. The sound should be audible and should be similar to the sound of the ocean.

Ujjayi breathing is said to have a calming effect on the nervous system and can help to focus the mind, making it a great technique for meditation. It can also help to improve lung capacity and can be beneficial for those with respiratory issues. Additionally, it can help to increase the internal heat of the body which can help to detoxify the body and increase flexibility in the muscles.

Nadi Shodhana (Alternate Nostril Breathing)

Nadi Shodhana, also known as "alternate nostril breathing," is a pranayama (breathing technique) used in yoga. It is a technique used to balance the energy flow in the body by alternating the breath between the left and right nostrils.

To practice Nadi Shodhana, sit in a comfortable position and use your right hand to close off your right nostril with your thumb, and inhale deeply through the left nostril. Then, use your ring finger to close off the left nostril and exhale through the right nostril. After exhaling, inhale through the right nostril, then exhale through the left. This completes one round of Nadi Shodhana.

Nadi Shodhana is said to have a calming effect on the mind and body, and it's believed to balance the left and right hemispheres of the brain. It's also said to help to balance the flow of prana (vital energy) throughout the body. Additionally, it can help to relieve stress and anxiety and improve concentration and focus. It's also said to be helpful for those who suffer from respiratory issues and improve lung capacity. It's a powerful and calming technique that can help to balance the body and mind, and is commonly used in yoga and meditation practices.

Kapalabhati (Skull Shining Breath)

Kapalabhati, also known as "skull shining breath," is a pranayama (breathing technique) used in yoga. It is a powerful, energizing breathing technique that involves rapid and forceful exhalations, followed by passive inhalations.

To practice Kapalabhati, sit in a comfortable position and take a deep breath in. Then, forcefully exhale through your nose, engaging your abdominal muscles to push the breath out. After exhaling, the breath should automatically flow back in passively. Repeat this rapid and forceful exhaling and passive inhaling, with the focus on the exhaling part. The breath should be smooth and even, with no pauses or jerks.

Kapalabhati is said to have a stimulating effect on the body and mind, and it's believed to increase energy levels and mental clarity. It's also said to help to purify the nasal passages, sinuses, and lungs. Additionally, it can help to strengthen the abdominal and respiratory muscles and improve digestion. It's also believed to balance energy and blood flow throughout the body. However, it's important to practice this technique under the guidance of an experienced teacher, as it can be intense and if not practiced correctly, it can cause strain on the body.

Building a Yoga Routine

To get the most out of your yoga practice, it is important to establish a regular routine. Start with a few minutes of yoga each day and gradually increase the time as you become more comfortable with the poses. Remember that consistency is key, and it's better to practice for a short time every day than to practice for a long time once a week.

With these basics in mind, you are ready to start your yoga practice. Remember to take your time, listen to your body, and be patient with yourself. With regular practice, you will see improvements in your flexibility, strength, and overall well-being.

Starting a yoga routine can be a great way to improve your physical and mental well-being, so here are some steps to help you get started:

1. **Set your intention:** Decide why you want to start practicing yoga and what you hope to gain from it. This can help you stay motivated and focused on your goals.

2. **Choose a style of yoga:** There are many different styles of yoga, each with its own focus and benefits. Research the different styles and choose one that appeals to you and aligns with your goals.

3. **Find a teacher:** If possible, attend a few classes with a qualified yoga instructor to learn the basics and ensure that you are practicing correctly and safely.

4. **Set aside time:** Decide on a regular time each day or each week to practice yoga. Make this time a priority and treat it as an appointment with yourself.

5. **Start slow:** Begin with a basic practice and gradually build up as you become more comfortable and confident. Focus on proper alignment and breathe deeply throughout each posture.

6. **Listen to your body:** Pay attention to your body and avoid pushing yourself too hard. Stop if you feel any pain or discomfort and never force yourself into a posture that feels unnatural.

7. **Incorporate meditation:** Meditation is an important aspect of yoga and can help you quiet your mind and reduce stress. Consider adding a few minutes of meditation to the end of your yoga practice.

8. **Be consistent:** To see the benefits of yoga, it's important to practice regularly. Try to stick to your routine and make yoga a regular part of your life.

Building a yoga routine takes time and dedication, but the rewards are well worth it. Start slow, listen to your body, and be consistent, and you'll soon see the benefits of a regular yoga practice.

Including Yoga Into Your Workout Routine

You can start a yoga routine even if you already have a workout routine, you could actually incorporate your yoga routine into your workout routine.

Incorporating yoga into your workout routine can be a great way to enhance your physical and mental well-being. Here are some tips for integrating yoga into your workout routine:

1. **Choose the right style:** Different styles of yoga will focus on different aspects of fitness, such as strength, flexibility, or balance. Consider your goals and choose a style of yoga that complements your existing workout routine.

2. **Warm up with yoga:** Use yoga as a warm-up before your other workout activities. This can help you to loosen up, improve flexibility, and get into a calm and focused mindset.

3. **Focus on balance:** Many yoga postures can help you improve your balance, which can have a positive impact on your other workouts. Incorporate balance postures, such as Tree Pose or Warrior III, into your routine.

4. **Use yoga for recovery:** Yoga can be an effective way to recover from other types of workouts, such as running or weightlifting. Consider incorporating restorative yoga or gentle yoga into your routine to help your body recover from intense workouts.

5. **Combine with cardio:** Some styles of yoga, such as vinyasa flow, can be very dynamic and provide an effective cardiovascular workout. Consider combining a yoga practice with other types of cardio, such as running or cycling, to get the best of both worlds.

6. **Incorporate meditation:** Yoga and meditation can be a powerful combination, and meditation can help you reduce stress and improve focus. Consider incorporating a few minutes of meditation into your routine after your yoga practice.

Incorporating yoga into your workout routine can bring many benefits, including improved flexibility, balance, and mental well-being. Choose a style of yoga that complements your existing routine, and focus on using yoga as a warm-up, recovery tool, and stress-reducer.

Incorporating Yoga Into Your Daily Life

To be able to carry on with your yoga routine on its own or during your workout, you need to turn your yoga practice into a habit. Making yoga a habit requires discipline and consistency, but the benefits are well worth it. Here are some tips to help you make yoga a habit:

1. **Make a commitment:** Make a conscious decision to prioritize yoga in your life and treat it as an important part of your daily routine.

2. **Find a convenient time:** Choose a time each day or each week to practice yoga that works well for your schedule and make it a non-negotiable part of your routine.

3. **Create a designated space:** Set up a dedicated space for your yoga practice, and make it comfortable and inviting. This can help you establish a connection with your practice and make it feel more special.

4. **Get an accountability partner:** Find someone who also wants to make yoga a habit and practice together. Having a partner can help you stay motivated and accountable.

5. **Set achievable goals:** Start with a basic practice and gradually increase the difficulty of your poses as you become more comfortable and confident. Setting achievable goals can help you see progress and stay motivated.

6. **Be consistent:** To make yoga a habit, it's important to practice regularly and consistently. Try to stick to your routine and avoid skipping sessions.

7. **Make it enjoyable:** Find ways to make your yoga practice enjoyable and fun. Consider incorporating

music, aromatherapy, or a special prop that you love into your practice.

8. **Celebrate your successes:** Take time to reflect on your progress and celebrate your successes, no matter how small. This can help you stay motivated and build a positive relationship with your yoga practice.

Making yoga a habit takes time and effort, but the benefits are well worth it. Prioritize your practice, make it convenient and enjoyable, and be consistent and you'll soon see the benefits of a regular yoga practice.

Chapter 3: Yoga for Health and Wellness

Yoga for Stress Relief

Yoga has been shown to be effective in reducing stress and anxiety. It can help to lower the levels of the stress hormone cortisol and increase the levels of the feel-good hormone serotonin. Yoga can also help to improve sleep and reduce symptoms of depression.

Yoga poses that are particularly effective for stress relief include:

Child's Pose

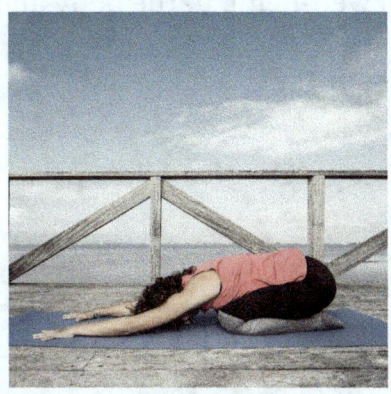

The Child's pose, also known as Balasana in Sanskrit, is a yoga pose that is often used as a resting pose between other yoga poses.

To perform Child's pose, start on your hands and knees, with your hands positioned directly under your shoulders and your knees positioned directly under your hips. Sit back on your heels and stretch your arms forward, with your palms facing down. Keep your head down and let your forehead rest on the mat. Hold this pose for as long as you are comfortable, breathing deeply and relaxing your entire body.

Child's pose is a gentle and restorative pose that can help to stretch the hips, thighs, and ankles. It's also said to calm the mind and relieve stress and anxiety. Additionally, it can help to relieve tension in the neck and back, making it a great pose for those with back pain. This pose is also often used in prenatal yoga, as it's considered a safe pose for pregnant women. Overall, Child's pose is a calming and grounding pose that can help to restore balance and well-being to the body and mind.

Legs-Up-the-Wall pose

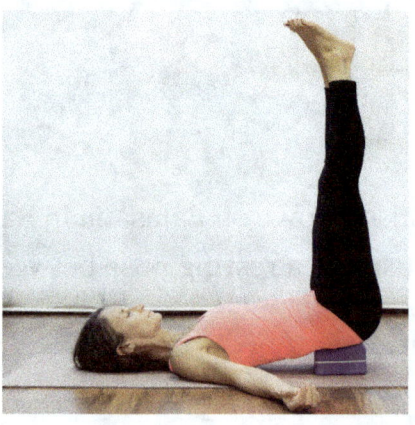

Legs-Up-the-Wall Pose, also known as Viparita Karani in Sanskrit, is a restorative yoga pose that can be used to relieve stress and fatigue, improve circulation, and calm the mind.

To perform Legs-Up-the-Wall Pose, start by sitting sideways against a wall, with your left hip closest to the wall. Then, swing your legs up onto the wall, so that your buttocks are resting against the wall and your legs are straight up in the air. You can place a pillow or blanket under your hips for additional support if needed. Allow your arms to rest by your sides, with your palms facing up. Hold this pose for as long as you are comfortable, breathing deeply and relaxing your entire body.

Legs-Up-the-Wall Pose is a gentle and restorative pose that can help to improve circulation, reduce swelling in the legs, and alleviate mild lower back pain. It's also said to be a calming and rejuvenating pose and can help to reduce stress and anxiety. Additionally, it's considered a safe and restorative pose for pregnant women, as it can help to alleviate discomfort and improve circulation. This pose is often used in restorative yoga practices and is a great way to end a yoga practice or unwind after a long day.

Corpse pose, which we already described in "Chapter 2 - The Foundations".

Alternate Nostril Breathing, also described in "Chapter 2 - Breathing Techniques".

Yoga for Flexibility and Strength

Yoga can help to improve flexibility and strength in the muscles and joints. It can help to increase the range of motion in the body and improve posture. Yoga poses that are particularly effective for building strength and flexibility include:

Downward-Facing Dog, which we already described in "Chapter 2 - The Foundations"

Warrior I and II

Warrior I Pose, also known as Virabhadrasana I in Sanskrit, is a standing yoga pose that strengthens the legs, hips, and core, and improves balance and stability.

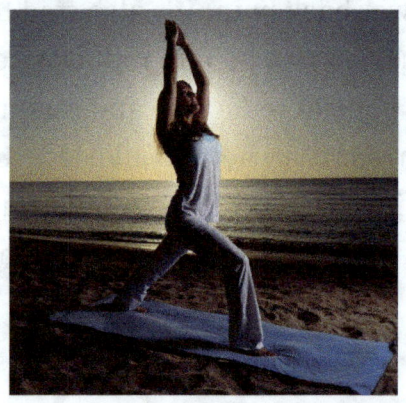

To perform Warrior I Pose, start in a standing position, with your feet hip-width apart. Step your left foot back, keeping your feet about 3-4 feet apart, with your left foot turned out to the side and your right foot facing forward. Bend your right knee and raise your arms above your head, with your palms facing each other. Make sure your right knee is directly over your ankle, and your left leg is straight. Gaze up towards your hands, and hold the pose for 5-10 breaths, breathing deeply and feeling the stretch in your hips and legs. Then, release the pose and repeat on the other side.

Warrior I Pose is a powerful and energizing pose that can help to improve strength and balance and is also said to be invigorating for the mind and body. Additionally, it can help to open the hips and chest and improve flexibility in the legs and hips. It's also a great pose for improving posture and core stability and is often used in sun salutation sequences and other dynamic yoga practices. Overall, the Warrior I Pose is a dynamic and energizing pose that can help to build strength and stability, both physically and mentally.

Warrior II Pose, also known as Virabhadrasana II in Sanskrit, is a standing yoga pose that strengthens the legs, hips, and core, and improves balance and stability.

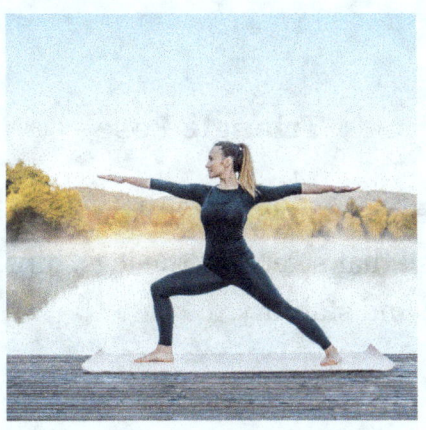

To perform Warrior II Pose, start in a standing position, with your feet hip-width apart. Step your left foot out to the side, about 3-4 feet apart, and turn your left foot out to the side. Bend your left knee and raise your arms out to the sides, with your left arm in front of your left leg and your right arm behind your back. Your left arm should be parallel to the ground and your right arm should be perpendicular to the ground. Gaze over your left fingertips and hold the pose for 5-10 breaths, breathing deeply and feeling the stretch in your hips and legs. Then, release the pose and repeat on the other side.

Warrior II Pose is a powerful and energizing pose that can help to improve strength and balance and is also said to be invigorating for the mind and body. Additionally, it can help to open the hips and chest and improve flexibility in the legs and hips. It's also a great pose for improving posture and core stability and is often used in sun salutation sequences and other dynamic yoga practices. Overall, Warrior II Pose is a dynamic and energizing pose that can help to build strength and stability, both physically and mentally.

Triangle Pose

The Triangle Pose, also known as Trikonasana in Sanskrit, is a standing yoga pose that stretches the legs, hips, and spine, and improves balance and stability.

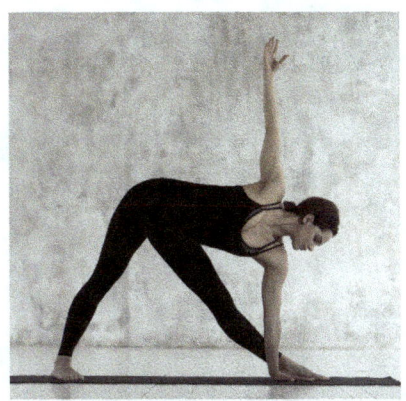

To perform Triangle Pose, start in a standing position, with your feet about 3-4 feet apart. Turn your right foot out to the side and your left foot in slightly towards the center. Reach your right hand down towards your right ankle and extend your left arm up towards the ceiling, with your palms facing each other. Make sure your legs are straight and your hips are facing forward, and hold the pose for 5-10 breaths, breathing deeply and feeling the stretch in your legs, hips, and spine. Then, release the pose and repeat on the other side.

Triangle Pose is a dynamic and energizing pose that can help to improve balance, stability, and flexibility, as well as stretch and open the hips, legs, and spine. Additionally, it's said to be calming for the mind and can help to relieve stress and anxiety. It's also a great pose for improving posture and core stability and is often used in sun salutation sequences and other dynamic yoga practices. Overall, Triangle Pose is a powerful and invigorating pose that can help to improve both physical and mental well-being.

Crow Pose

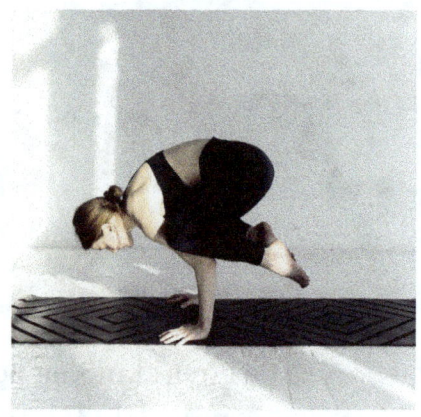

Crow Pose, also known as Bakasana in Sanskrit, is an arm-balancing yoga pose that strengthens the arms, wrists, and core, and improves balance and stability.

To perform Crow Pose, start in a squatting position, with your knees wider than hip-width apart and your hands on the ground in front of you. Place your hands shoulder-width apart, with your fingers spread wide and your fingertips pointing forward. Lean forward, keeping your weight over your arms, and lift your feet off the ground, bringing your knees into your arms. Keep your gaze forward and focus on finding your balance. Hold the pose for 5-10 breaths, breathing deeply and feeling the strengthening in your arms, wrists, and core.

Crow Pose is a challenging and empowering pose that can help to build strength and stability, both physically and mentally. Additionally, it's said to be invigorating for the mind and can help to boost confidence and focus. It's also a great pose for improving balance and coordination and is often used in more advanced yoga sequences and practices. Overall, Crow Pose is a dynamic and strengthening pose that can help to build both physical and mental strength and stability.

Yoga for Cardiovascular Health

Yoga can also have a positive impact on cardiovascular health. It can help to lower blood pressure and improve circulation and cardiovascular fitness. Yoga poses that are particularly effective for cardiovascular health include:

Sun Salutation

Sun Salutation, also known as Surya Namaskar in Sanskrit, is a series of yoga poses performed in a flowing sequence to warm up the body and mind, improve flexibility and balance, and build strength and stability.

A typical Sun Salutation sequence consists of 12 poses that are performed in a specific order.

The correct order of the twelve poses in a Sun Salutation sequence is:

1. **Mountain Pose** (Tadasana) (see "Chapter 2 - The Foundations")

2. **Raised Arms Pose** (Urdhva Hastasana) (see description below)

3. **Forward Bend** (Uttanasana) (see "Chapter 2 - the Foundations")

4. **Lunge Pose** (Anjaneyasana) (see description below)

5. **Four-Limbed Staff Pose** (Chaturanga Dandasana) (see description below)

6. **Cobra Pose** (Bhujangasana) (see "Chapter 2 - The Foundations")

7. **Downward-Facing Dog Pose** (Adho Mukha Svanasana) (see "Chapter 2 - The Foundations")

8. **Forward Bend** (Uttanasana) (see "Chapter 2 - The Foundations")

9. **Lunge Pose** (Anjaneyasana) (see description below)

10. **Raised Arms Pose** (Urdhva Hastasana) (see description below)

11. **Mountain Pose** (Tadasana) (see "Chapter 2 - The Foundations")

12. **Upward-Facing Dog Pose** (Urdhva Mukha Svanasana) (see "Chapter 2 - The Foundations")

The sequence is typically performed in a continuous, flowing movement, with each pose flowing smoothly into the next. The Sun Salutation is often used as a warm-up for yoga practice and is also used to build strength and flexibility, improve balance and coordination, and clear the mind and body.

Most of the poses that compose the sequence are already described in other chapters of the book look for them in case you need to refresh your mind on how to perform them. However, there are three poses' missing descriptions that I will list here.

The **Raised Arms Pose**, also known as Hasta Uttanasana in Sanskrit, is a simple standing yoga pose that can help to energize the body, stretch the muscles, and improve posture.

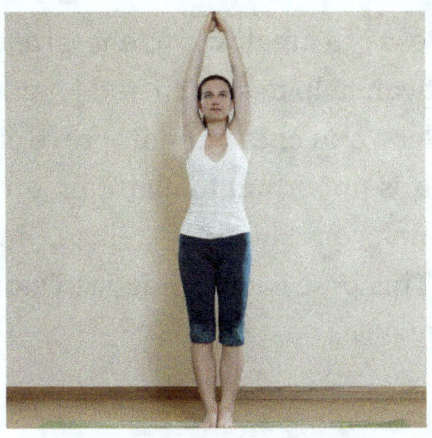

To perform the Raised Arms Pose:

1. Begin standing in Tadasana (Mountain Pose) with your feet hip-distance apart and your arms resting at your sides.

2. As you inhale, slowly raise your arms up and overhead, keeping your palms facing each other and your shoulders relaxed.

3. Stretch your arms upward as far as you comfortably can, keeping your gaze forward and your neck relaxed.

4. Take a few deep breaths in this position, feeling the stretch in your arms, chest, and shoulders.

5. As you exhale, lower your arms back down to your sides.

6. Repeat the pose for several rounds, inhaling as you raise your arms, and exhaling as you lower them back down.

The Raised Arms Pose is a great way to energize the body and improve posture. It can help to stretch and lengthen the muscles in the arms, shoulders, and chest, and improve circulation and breath awareness. It is important to maintain proper alignment in this pose by keeping your shoulders relaxed and your neck in a neutral position. This pose can be practiced alone or as a part of a larger yoga sequence.

The **Lunge Pose**, also known as Anjaneyasana in Sanskrit, is a common yoga pose that can help to stretch and strengthen the legs, hips, and lower back. It is often used as a transitional pose between other standing poses.

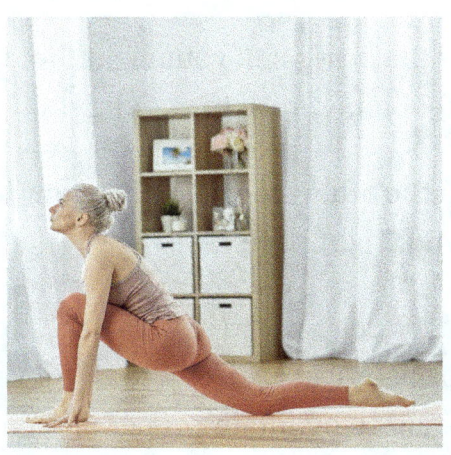

To perform the Lunge Pose:

1. Begin in a standing position at the front of your mat with your feet hip-distance apart.

2. Step your right foot back, placing the ball of your foot on the ground and extending your leg straight behind you.

3. Bend your left knee, bringing it directly over your ankle and lowering your hips toward the ground.

4. Place your hands on the ground on either side of your left foot, or keep your hands on your hips.

5. Lift your chest and gaze forward, keeping your shoulders relaxed and your neck in a neutral position.

6. Take a few deep breaths in this position, feeling the stretch in your legs and hips.

7. To release the pose, step your right foot forward to meet your left foot and return to standing.

8. Repeat on the other side, stepping your left foot back and bending your right knee.

The Lunge Pose is a great way to stretch and strengthen the legs, hips, and lower back. It can also help to improve balance and focus. It is important to maintain proper alignment in this pose by keeping your front knee directly over your ankle and your back leg extended straight behind you. If you have knee or hip injuries, it is important to consult with a yoga teacher or healthcare professional before practicing this pose.

The **Four-Limbed Staff Pose**, also known as Chaturanga Dandasana in Sanskrit, is a challenging yoga pose that is often used as a transition between the Plank Pose and the Upward-Facing Dog Pose. It can help to build strength in the arms, wrists, and core, as well as improve overall body awareness and alignment.

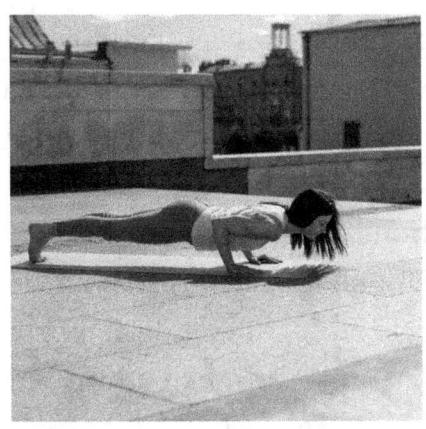

To perform the Four-Limbed Staff Pose:

1. Begin in the Plank Pose, with your hands and feet on the ground and your body in a straight line.

2. Lower your body down towards the ground, keeping your elbows close to your ribs and your shoulders away from your ears.

3. Stop when your arms are at a 90-degree angle, hovering just above the ground.

4. Keep your legs straight and engaged, and your core active to support your body.

5. Hold the pose for a few breaths, then release by either lowering all the way to the ground or pushing up to the Upward-Facing Dog Pose.

It's important to maintain proper alignment in this pose by keeping your elbows close to your ribs, your shoulders away from your ears, and your core engaged. If you're new to this pose, it's recommended to practice with your knees on the ground until you build enough strength to support your full body weight. The Four-Limbed Staff Pose is a challenging pose that can help to build strength, but it's important to listen to your body and avoid overexertion or strain.

Overall, Sun Salutation is a powerful and invigorating yoga practice that can help to build strength and stability, both physically and mentally, and is a great way to warm up the body and mind before a yoga practice or workout.

Here are the pictures of each pose of the sequence in the correct order of performance.

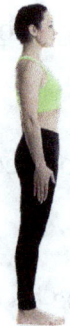 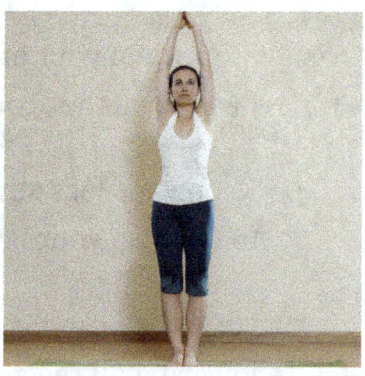

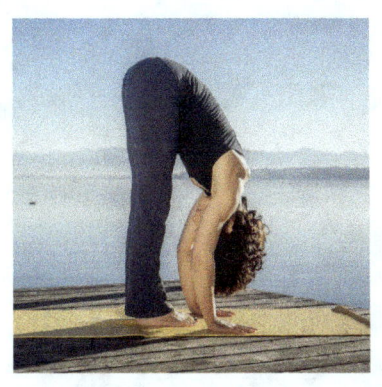
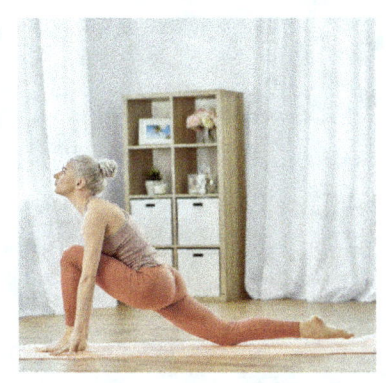
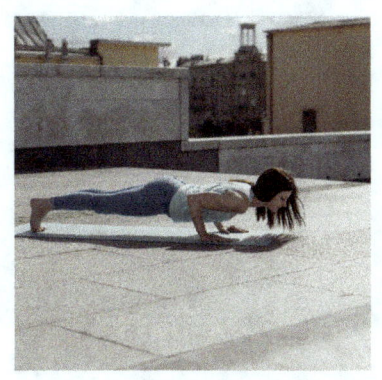
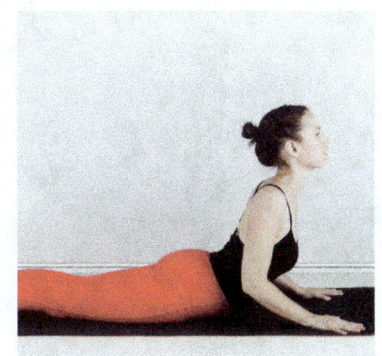
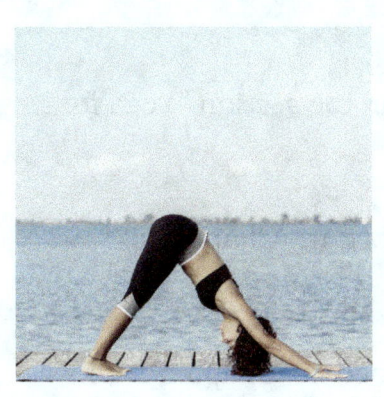
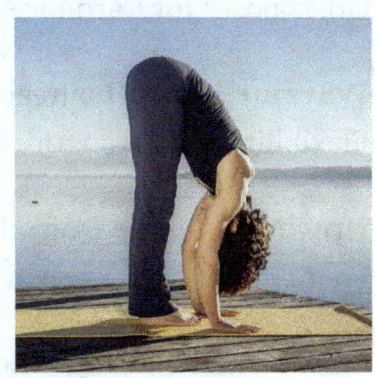

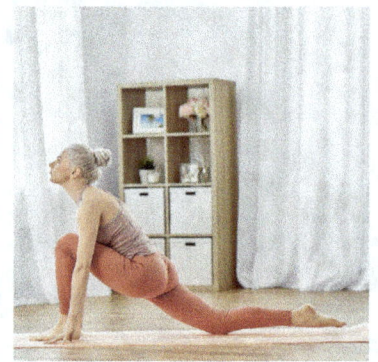 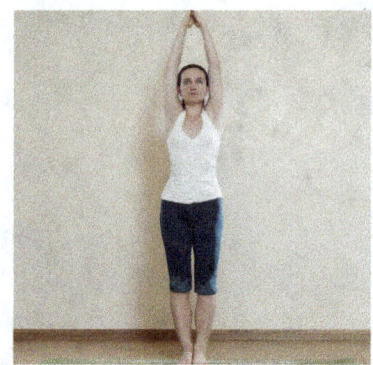

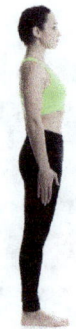 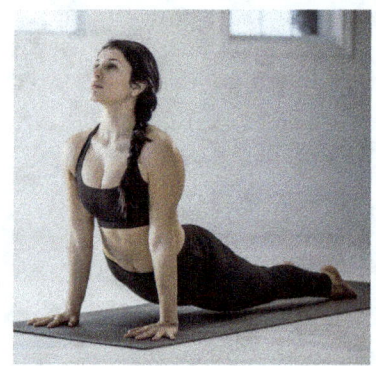

Other poses for Cardiovascular Health:

Warrior I and II, already described in the section "Yoga for Flexibility and Strength"

Upward-Facing Dog, already described in "Chapter 2 -The Foundations"

Downward-Facing Dog, also described in "Chapter 2 -The Foundations"

Yoga for Mental Health

Yoga has been shown to be effective in improving mental health. It can help to reduce symptoms of depression and anxiety and improve mood and overall sense of well-being. Yoga poses that are particularly effective for mental health include:

Child's Pose, already described in the section "Yoga for Stress Relief"

Corpse Pose, already described in in "Chapter 2 -The Foundations"

Seated Forward Bend

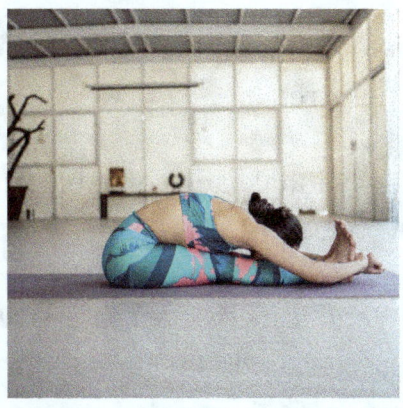

The Seated Forward Bend, also known as Paschimottanasana in Sanskrit, is a yoga pose that targets the hamstrings, lower back, and spine.

To perform this pose:

1. Begin seated on the mat with your legs extended straight out in front of you.

2. Sit up tall, with your back straight and your shoulders relaxed.

3. Breathe in and raise your arms up overhead.

4. Breathe out and hinge forward from your hips, reaching forward to grab hold of your toes or the soles of your feet.

5. Hold onto your feet and keep your spine long and straight as you gently fold forward.

6. Hold the pose for several breaths, breathing deeply and relaxing into the stretch.

7. To release, slowly inhale and come back up to a seated position, with your arms overhead.

The Seated Forward Bend is a great pose for stretching the hamstrings and lower back, and for calming the mind and body. It is also an excellent pose for improving posture, increasing flexibility, and reducing stress and tension.

Meditation is a huge subject you will find described in depth in my two previous books "Chakras" e "Meditation for Beginners". I already discussed part of the relationship between yoga and meditation in the previous chapters. However, yoga and meditation in conjunction have been shown to have many benefits for mental health which I would like to underline, including:

1. Reducing Stress: Both yoga and meditation have been shown to lower stress levels by reducing the levels of cortisol, the stress hormone, in the body.

2. Improving Mood: Regular practice of yoga and meditation has been shown to increase positive emotions such as happiness, calmness, and inner peace, as well as reduce symptoms of anxiety, depression, and stress.

3. Enhancing Self-Awareness: Through the practice of yoga and meditation, people can gain a greater understanding of themselves and their thoughts, which can lead to increased self-awareness, self-esteem, and self-confidence.

4. Boosting Concentration: By training the mind to focus on the present moment, yoga and meditation can improve mental clarity and concentration, making it easier to stay focused and productive in daily life.

5. Promoting Relaxation: Both yoga and meditation help promote deep relaxation and calmness, which can be beneficial for people with sleep issues and insomnia.

6. Improving Cognitive Function: Some studies have shown that regular practice of yoga and meditation can help

improve cognitive function, including memory, reasoning, and perception.

Overall, yoga and meditation offer several benefits for mental health and can be an effective complement to traditional mental health treatments such as therapy and medication. However, it's important to note that if you're experiencing symptoms of a mental health condition, you should always consult with a mental health professional.

Yoga for Weight Management

Yoga can also be helpful for weight management. It can help to boost metabolism and increase muscle mass, which can aid in weight loss. Additionally, yoga can help to reduce stress and improve overall well-being, which can also aid in weight loss. Yoga poses that are particularly effective for weight management include:

Sun Salutation, already described in the section "Yoga for Cardiovascular Health"

Warrior I and II, already described in the section "Yoga for Flexibility and Strength"

Triangle Pose, already described in the section "Yoga for Flexibility and Strength"

Crow Pose, already described in the section "Yoga for Flexibility and Strength"

Remember to consult with your physician before starting any new exercise program if you have any health concerns.

Chapter 4: Yoga for Special Populations

Yoga for Seniors

Yoga can be a great form of exercise for seniors. It can help to improve flexibility, strength, balance, and cardiovascular health. Additionally, yoga can help to reduce stress and improve overall well-being. Yoga poses that are particularly beneficial for seniors include:

Mountain Pose, already described in "Chapter 2 -The Foundations"

Standing Forward Bend, already described in "Chapter 2 -The Foundations"

Cobra Pose, already described in "Chapter 2 -The Foundations"

Locust Pose

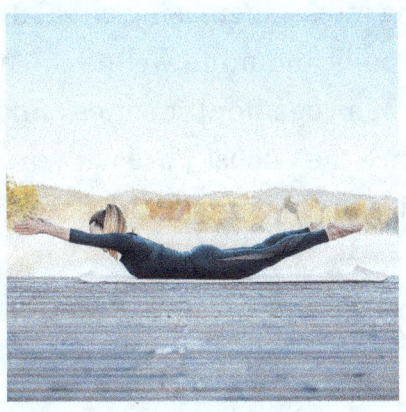

The Locust Pose, also known as Salabhasana in Sanskrit, is a yoga pose that strengthens the back muscles and stretches the spine, chest, and legs.

To perform the Locust Pose:

1. Lie on your stomach with your arms along your sides, legs extended straight behind you, and your chin resting on the floor.

2. Inhale, and lift your head, arms, legs, and upper body off the ground. Keep your arms straight, your legs close together, and your feet pointing straight back.

3. Hold the pose for a few breaths, focusing on the stretch in your back, legs, and arms.

4. To release, exhale and lower yourself back down to the ground.

The Locust Pose is a great pose for strengthening the back muscles, stretching the spine, and improving posture. It is also helpful for reducing stress, increasing circulation, and promoting overall body and mind wellness. This pose is typically performed as part of a yoga flow or series of poses. It is important to practice the Locust Pose with proper form to avoid injury and maximize the benefits of the pose.

Corpse Pose, already described in "Chapter 2 -The Foundations"

Yoga for Children

Yoga can also be beneficial for children. It can help to improve flexibility, strength, and balance, as well as reduce stress and anxiety. Yoga poses that are particularly beneficial for children include:

Child's Pose, already described in the section "Yoga for Stress Relief"

Downward-Facing Dog, already described in "Chapter 2 -The Foundations"

Warrior I and II, already described in the section "Yoga for Flexibility and Strength"

Tree Pose

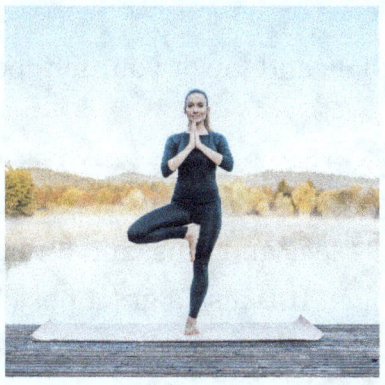

The Tree Pose, also known as Vrksasana in Sanskrit, is a yoga pose that helps improve balance, stability, and focus while stretching the legs and hips.

To perform the Tree Pose:

1. Begin standing with your feet hip-width apart and your hands on your hips.

2. Shift your weight onto your right foot and bend your left knee.

3. Place the sole of your left foot on the inside of your right thigh, keeping your left knee pointed out to the side.

4. Press your foot into your thigh and bring your hands to prayer position at your chest.

5. If you feel stable, raise your arms above your head, keeping your palms touching.

6. Hold the pose for a few breaths, focusing on your balance and breathing.

7. To release, exhale and lower your left foot back to the ground.

The Tree Pose is a great pose for improving balance and stability, stretching the legs and hips, and building strength in the legs, ankles, and feet. It is also a great pose for reducing stress, improving focus, and promoting overall body and mind wellness. It is important to practice the Tree Pose with proper form to avoid injury and maximize the benefits of the pose.

-Savasana (Corpse Pose), already described in "Chapter 2 -The Foundations"

Yoga for Pregnant Women

Yoga can be a great form of exercise for pregnant women. It can help to improve flexibility, strength, and balance. Additionally, yoga can help to reduce stress and improve overall well-being. Yoga poses that are particularly beneficial for pregnant women include:

Cat-Cow Pose

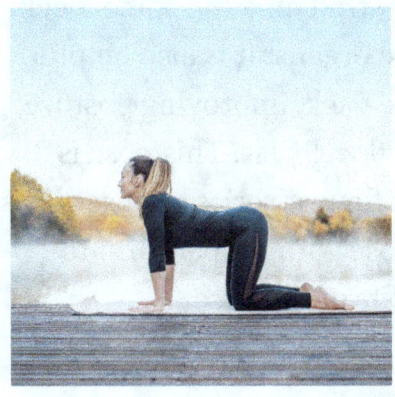 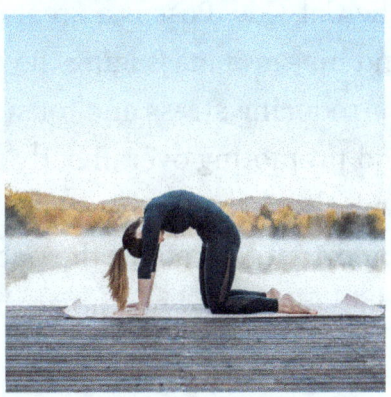

The Cat-Cow Pose, also known as Marjaryasana-Bitilasana in Sanskrit, is a yoga pose that helps to stretch the spine, neck, and hips while massaging the digestive organs and increasing flexibility in the back.

To perform the Cat-Cow Pose:

1. Start on your hands and knees, with your wrists directly under your shoulders and your knees under your hips.

2. As you inhale, drop your belly towards the ground, lifting your head and tailbone up towards the ceiling, creating a gentle arch in your back. This is the Cow Pose.

3. As you exhale, round your spine towards the ceiling, tucking your chin to your chest and tucking your tailbone under. This is the Cat Pose.

4. Repeat the movement, flowing smoothly between the Cow Pose and the Cat Pose for several breaths.

The Cat-Cow Pose is a great pose for stretching the spine, neck, and hips and massaging the digestive organs. It is also helpful for reducing stress and tension in the back, improving posture, and promoting overall body and mind wellness. This pose is typically performed as part of a yoga flow or series of poses. It is important to practice the Cat-Cow Pose with proper form to avoid injury and maximize the benefits of the pose.

Downward-Facing Dog, already described in "Chapter 2 -The Foundations"

Warrior I and II, already described in the section "Yoga for Flexibility and Strength"

Child's Pose, already described in the section "Yoga for Stress Relief"

Corpse Pose, already described in "Chapter 2 -The Foundations"

Yoga for Athletes

Yoga can also be beneficial for athletes. It can help to improve flexibility, strength, and balance, as well as reduce stress and anxiety. Yoga poses that are particularly beneficial for athletes include:

Downward-Facing Dog, already described in "Chapter 2 -The Foundations"

Warrior I and II, already described in the section "Yoga for Flexibility and Strength"

Crow Pose, already described in the section "Yoga for Flexibility and Strength"

Pigeon Pose

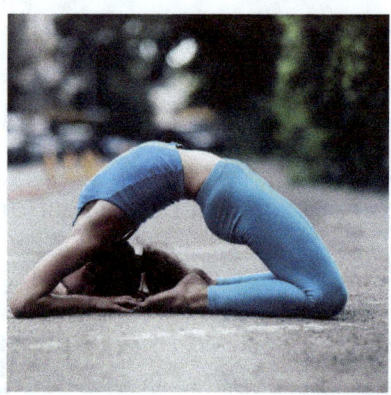

The Pigeon Pose, also known as Kapotasana in Sanskrit, is a yoga pose that helps to stretch the hips, thighs, and lower back, while also opening up the hips and releasing tension in the hips and lower back.

To perform the Pigeon Pose:

1. Begin in a Downward-Facing Dog Pose.

2. Bring your right knee to your right hand and place your right ankle near your left wrist.

3. Slowly lower your right knee to the ground and extend your left leg behind you, keeping your left knee and foot pointing straight up towards the ceiling.

4. Use your hands to support yourself on either side of your hips, or lower your torso to the ground.

5. Hold the pose for several breaths, focusing on your breath and the stretch in your hips and lower back.

6. To release, push into your hands or arms and slowly straighten your right leg, returning to the Downward-Facing Dog Pose.

7. Repeat the pose on the other side.

The Pigeon Pose is a great pose for stretching the hips, thighs, and lower back, and for opening up the hips and releasing tension in the hips and lower back. It is also helpful for improving hip flexibility, reducing stress and tension in the hips and lower back, and promoting overall body and mind wellness. It is important to practice the Pigeon Pose with proper form to avoid injury and maximize the benefits of the pose.

Corpse Pose, already described in "Chapter 2 -The Foundations"

Yoga for People with Chronic Conditions

Yoga can be beneficial for people with chronic conditions such as arthritis, fibromyalgia, and back pain. It can help to improve flexibility, strength, and balance, as well as reduce stress and anxiety. Yoga poses that are particularly beneficial for people with chronic conditions include:

Child's Pose, already described in the section "Yoga for Stress Relief"

Cat-Cow Pose, already described in the section "Yoga for Pregnant Woman"

Downward-Facing Dog, already described in "Chapter 2 -The Foundations"

Warrior I and II, already described in the section "Yoga for Flexibility and Strength"

Corpse Pose, already described in "Chapter 2 -The Foundations"

It is important to consult with a physician before starting a yoga practice if you have any chronic conditions. Additionally, it is best to seek out a qualified yoga teacher who has experience working with people with your specific condition.

Chapter 5: Misunderstandings and False Beliefs About Yoga

There are certainly false beliefs and misunderstandings about yoga. Some of the most common misconceptions about yoga include:

1. **Yoga is just stretching:** While yoga does involve physical postures that stretch the body, it is much more than just a form of exercise. Yoga encompasses a wide range of practices, including breath control, meditation, and self-reflection, that are designed to bring balance and harmony to the mind, body, and spirit.

2. **Yoga is a religion:** Yoga is not a religion and does not require any specific belief system. However, it is deeply rooted in the spiritual traditions of Hinduism and Buddhism and may incorporate elements of spirituality or philosophy that are meaningful to practitioners.

3. **Yoga is only for women:** This is a false stereotype and is not reflective of the diversity of yoga practitioners. Yoga is for people of all genders, ages, and abilities, and can be adapted to meet the needs of each individual.

4. **Yoga is easy:** While some yoga postures may look simple, they can be surprisingly challenging and require a great deal of strength, flexibility, and focus. Yoga is not

an easy practice and requires dedication and effort to master.

5. **Yoga is only about physical postures:** While the physical practice of yoga is important, it is just one aspect of this multi-faceted discipline. Yoga also includes breath control, meditation, and ethical principles, all of which work together to bring balance and harmony to the mind, body, and spirit.

6. **Yoga is only for the flexible:** Flexibility is not a requirement to begin practicing yoga. In fact, many people start practicing yoga because they want to improve their flexibility, and the practice itself can help increase flexibility over time.

7. **Yoga is only for the young and healthy:** Yoga is a practice that can be adapted to meet the needs of people of all ages and abilities. Whether you are young or old, fit or not, there is a type of yoga that can be beneficial for you.

8. **Yoga is expensive:** While some yoga studios and retreats can be expensive, there are many affordable and even free resources available for those who want to practice yoga. From online videos to community classes, there are many ways to start practicing yoga without breaking the bank.

9. **Yoga is a cure-all:** While yoga can offer many benefits, it is not a cure-all and should not be used as a substitute for medical treatment. It is always a good idea to consult with your doctor before starting a new exercise routine, especially if you have any medical conditions.

It's important to remember that yoga is a personal practice, and each individual's experience with yoga will be unique. By approaching yoga with an open mind and a willingness to learn, you can begin to uncover its many benefits and dispel any false beliefs or misconceptions you may have about the practice.

Conclusion

Tips for a Successful Yoga Practice

- Start with a few minutes of yoga each day and gradually increase the time as you become more comfortable with the poses.

- Remember to take your time and listen to your body.

- Be patient with yourself and don't expect to be able to do all the poses right away.

- Find a qualified teacher who can guide you through the correct alignment and modifications.

- Practice in a quiet, distraction-free space.

- Remember to breathe deeply and focus on your breath.

Warnings

Here are a few things to keep in mind before starting a yoga practice:

1. **Consult with your doctor:** If you have any medical conditions, it is always a good idea to consult with your doctor before starting a new exercise routine, especially if you have a history of injury or medical concerns.

2. **Start with a beginner class:** If you are new to yoga, it is important to start with a beginner class to learn the basics of the practice and ensure you are performing the poses safely and correctly.

3. **Be patient with yourself:** Yoga can be a challenging practice, both physically and mentally, but it is important to be patient with yourself and not compare yourself to others in your class. Focus on your own progress and don't get discouraged if you can't perform a pose perfectly at first.

4. **Listen to your body:** Yoga is a low-impact practice, but it can still be physically demanding. It is important to listen to your body and stop or modify a pose if you experience pain or discomfort.

5. **Focus on proper alignment:** Proper alignment is important in yoga to prevent injury and ensure you are getting the most out of each pose. Take the time to learn

the proper alignment and focus on it during your practice.

6. **Find a teacher you trust:** A good yoga teacher can make all the difference in your practice. Look for a teacher who is knowledgeable, experienced, and who you feel comfortable with that can help you getting started.

7. **Respect your limitations:** Yoga is a practice that should be adapted to meet your individual needs and limitations. Don't push yourself too hard or try to perform poses that are beyond your ability. Instead, focus on finding modifications that work for you and respect your limitations.

Glossary of Yoga Terms

- **Asana:** physical postures

- **Dharana:** concentration

- **Dhyana:** meditation

- **Mantra:** a word or phrase repeated during meditation

- **Mudra:** hand gestures used during meditation

- **Namaste:** a traditional yoga greeting

- **Pranayama:** breath control

- **Samadhi:** the state of unity with the divine

- **Sanskrit:** the ancient language of India in which many yoga texts are written

- **Yama:** ethical guidelines for behavior towards others

The Path to Total Wellness & Recommended Reading

As you have learned throughout this book, yoga offers a wealth of benefits for the body, mind, and spirit. By incorporating a regular yoga practice into your daily routine, you can increase strength and flexibility, reduce stress and anxiety, and cultivate a deeper sense of inner peace and happiness.

However, to fully experience the transformative power of yoga, it is essential to have a comprehensive understanding of the various aspects that make up this ancient practice. This includes not only the physical postures but also the spiritual and energetic aspects that are intertwined with each movement.

That is why I strongly recommend that you continue your journey of self-discovery and growth by reading my two previous books, "Chakras for Beginners" by Mind, Body, and Spirit Masterclass (ISBN: 9781739665210) and "Meditation for Beginners" by Mind, Body, and Spirit Masterclass (ISBN: 9781739665234). These books delve deeper into the chakra system and meditation practices, respectively, and will give you a complete picture of the holistic approach to wellness that yoga offers.

Remember to take your time, listen to your body, and be patient with yourself. With regular practice, you will see improvements in your flexibility, strength, and overall well-being.

By combining the physical, spiritual, and energetic aspects of yoga, you will be able to truly unlock its full potential and achieve a state of total wellness. So I encourage you to take the next step and continue your exploration of this amazing practice. I hope that this book has provided you with a solid foundation for your yoga practice.

Namaste

Anja D.

www.ingramcontent.com/pod-product-compliance
Lightning Source LLC
Chambersburg PA
CBHW050305120526
44590CB00016B/2503